Dodging Diabetes Deliciously can change your life. These recipes are not only scrumptious, they are soulful. The pictures and words in this book show cooking as an act of love and creativity. By learning to care for your body's long-term needs, you can make eating less anxiety provoking and more fun. You may not be able to have your cake and eat it too, but you can nourish your body, soul and appetite all at once.

— JODI HALPERN, M.D., Ph.D.,
UC Berkeley Joint Medical Program and School of Public Health
author of *From Detached Concern to Empathy: Humanizing Medical Practice*

Diabetes remains one of the most insidious health issues in America. We must take back control of our own health and be less dependent on drug companies. I was overjoyed to find this realistic, practical cookbook for those with prediabetes. This approach is refreshing, and the recipes are uncomplicated. Hats off to Drs. Holmes and Snider for their most savory and helpful piece of culinary work!

— MELVIN J. HUIE, M.D.,
Internal Medicine, Orinda, CA

What an empowering book! *Dodging Diabetes Deliciously* will help regulate your blood sugar and introduce you to wonderful food designed to satiate and nourish you toward vibrant health. Taste and flavor make these sumptuous and satisfying dishes memorable. The recipes included within these pages will become an important part of your culinary canon.

— REBECCA KATZ, M.S.,
author of *The Longevity Kitchen: Satisfying, Big-Flavor Recipes*
Featuring the Top 16 Age-Busting Power Foods*

The explosion of type 2 diabetes is the most important public health issue facing developed countries today. One in every three adults in the United States has prediabetes. These appetizing, easy recipes undoubtedly will help many to either cure the condition or prevent progression to full-blown diabetes. I wish all my prediabetic patients would read this book and put its principles into practice. I highly recommend *Dodging Diabetes Deliciously* for anyone with prediabetes.

— STEVE PARKER, M.D.,
author of *Conquer Diabetes and Prediabetes: The Low-Carb Mediterranean Diet*

This book is the best guide I've seen for celebrating the delights of low-carb, healthy and delectable cooking. Enjoy!

— DONNA CHAMBERLAIN, B.S.,
Co-founder, *Maine Cottage Foods LLC*

Excellent! *Dodging Diabetes Deliciously* employs diabetes science and offers strategies and exciting recipes that fit the science perfectly. The coherent organization of specialized recipes will make *DDD* an enduring culinary guide to diabetic-friendly family dinners and entertaining. Get it, read it, learn from it, love it!

— ARLENE SEMERJIAN, Ph.D.,
Co-founder, *Maine Cottage Foods LLC*

DODGING DIABETES DELICIOUSLY

A Low-Carb Approach to Prediabetes

Constance Holmes, Ed.D.
Martha Snider, M.D.

REGENT PRESS
Berkeley, California

[paperback book]
ISBN 13: 978-1-58790-252-9
ISBN 10: 1-58790-252-4

[e-book]
ISBN 13: 978-1-58790-253-6
ISBN 10: 1-58790-253-2

Library of Congress Number: 2013951957

DISCLAIMER

The ideas and suggestions in this book are provided as general educational information only and should not be construed as medical advice or care. All matters regarding your health require supervision by a personal physician or other appropriate health professional familiar with your current health status. Always consult your personal physician before making any dietary, medication, or exercise changes. The publisher and authors disclaim any liability or warranties of any kind arising directly or indirectly from the use of this book. If any problems develop, always consult your personal physician. Only your physician can provide you medical advice.

REGENT PRESS
Berkeley, California
www.regentpress.net
regentpress@mindspring.com

For our mothers,
Margaret and Martha,
who were the first
to feed us.

For Mary Lynn,
in appreciation
and with admiration,

Anne Holmes

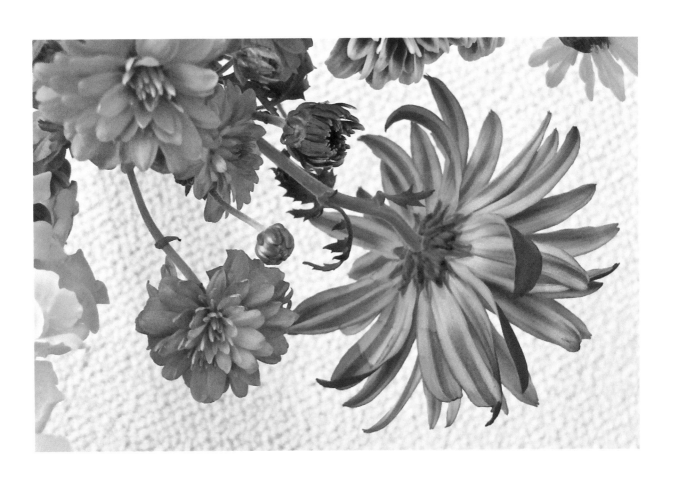

ACKNOWLEDGEMENTS & SPECIAL THANKS

To Sheila Boniface, Jesper Rosenmeier, Leslie Sanders and Brenda Vaccaro
for invaluable editing.
Thanks to Carlene St. John for her careful reading.

And *in memoriam* — Patricia Dacey, diabetic food lover and plucky supporter
and Lenore Lefer, wonderful cook, muse, ally and witness.

We have had some excellent taste testers for this cookbook. Many thanks to
Eliot Davidoff, Michael Graham, Jean Kilbourne, Stephanie Ng and Amalia Wille.

C.H.

Special thanks to Joan Bobkoff who has supported my work as a photographer
in many ways. Her ability to look at a body of work and perceive its strengths and
notice subtle themes is a gift she shares readily.

To my fellow writers, Johnnye Jones Gibson and Jodi Halpern,
thank you for your on-going support for this and every project
I've undertaken in the past three years.

Readers Judy Adler, Alison Aronstam, Sheila Boniface, Rebecca Brook,
Lea Delpomo, Charlene Echols, Joan Fierer, and Brenda Vaccaro
provided thoughtful and clarifying editorial suggestions.

To Mark Weiman, thank you for your encouragement, patience and for sharing
your knowledge about the business side of books.

Lastly, to fellow foodies, excellent cooks, and favorite dining companions
Eliot Davidoff and Amalia Wille, my heartfelt thanks!

M.S.

Introduction

by Constance Holmes, Ed.D.

I have always loved food. My mother delights in reporting that my first word was *more*. I haven't just loved food; I've been fascinated by it. Being in the kitchen, watching food being prepared, has always been my favorite entertainment. At a restaurant, I'm the diner who wants to know, not only ingredients, but exactly how my dish has been prepared.

Food and cooking have been a source of joy as well as a source of anxiety. Beginning in adolescence, I have struggled with weight gain — followed by weight loss — only to begin the cycle again. At age 12, I was put on my first high-protein, low-carbohydrate weight loss program and remember bringing sandwiches to school wrapped in lettuce leaves rather than slices of bread. As long as I stuck to a drastically carbohydrate-reduced food plan, I was able, with effort, to keep my weight at a healthier level. When I rejoined my more normal peers in eating carbohydrate-rich foods, my weight soared and my self-esteem plummeted.

Nevertheless, my interest and love of food remained constant. The imagination and invention involved in food design, creation and presentation captured me as a child. As an adult, I've been inspired by cooking as creation: how to coax the greatest flavor and deliciousness from the meal components before me.

Three years ago, I was diagnosed with prediabetes and I came to understand the role genetics plays in diabetes. My father was diagnosed with diabetes at age 45 and died of heart disease at age 60. His father, his brother and their grandfather had diabetes. My own diagnosis (not yet full-blown diabetes and still reversible) did not come as a shock given this genetic history, but I did need to face the truth of my situation. As my doctor put it, I am seriously glucose-intolerant which means I need to eat within strictly carbohydrate controlled limits.

Now I know how I need to eat in order to dodge diabetes. When I have added grain, root vegetables and tropical fruits back into my diet, my weight has gradually climbed. Facing the reality and permanence of this state has been strangely liberating. In addition, I need to be sure to make intense exercise a regular and happy part of my life. No longer bargaining with a "taste" of bread, mashed potatoes or dessert, I have opened my mind to the possibility of eating well, even deliciously, within limitations. I have received a lot of help in doing so, especially from my co-author, Martha Snider. Our book is the fruit of this exploration.

Finally fully aware of my situation, I decided to create a new way to cook and to eat. I needed a food life that supported my health, kept me clear of diabetes and yet retained all the deliciousness my body and soul required.

From Dr. Richard Bernstein, in *The Diabetes Solution*, I learned exactly how carbohydrates affect the metabolism of people like me with glucose intolerance and/or insulin resistance. Dr. Bernstein convinced me that everyone, including everyone being treated for diabetes, can have normal blood sugar if they stringently limit their daily carbohydrate intake to 45 grams or less. I learned that only protein and fat are without carbohydrates. Legumes, nuts, seeds, dairy products (except full-fat dairy), vegetables (especially root vegetables and winter squashes) and all fruits (especially tropical fruits and even apples) have carbohydrates that must be carefully counted in order to stay under that 45 gram bar.

Dr. Bernstein does have some good news. Delicious salad greens like arugula, endive, and mesclun are fairly low in carbs; so are asparagus, avocado, cauliflower, string beans, summer squashes, broccoli and bell peppers (except yellow ones). Brussels sprouts (among my favorite vegetables) can be roasted, braised, or steamed to delicious effect. Berries, among nature's most delicious morsels, are also mercifully low. And there are surprises: almond milk is very low in carbs and can be blended with frozen berries to create a toothsome sorbet.

Hard cheese is also fairly low in carbs although it is rich in calories. But a small amount of English Stilton (I recently savored it with thin slices of apple) makes for a scrumptious end to a meal. Goat cheese Brie served warm enough to ooze is a great treat especially with a few ripe cherries.

Rather than grimly focusing on what I needed to eliminate, I began to look to what I could eat safely. And I began to imagine what meals I could create from low-carb ingredients that would keep the count under 20 grams per meal.

Soon I was up against my love of chocolate. Recent studies lauding the benefits of dark chocolate as an anti-oxidant and a potential cancer fighter further reinforced my wish to include chocolate in my food life. Finding the best low-sugar, low-glycemic chocolatier online proved to be a demanding project. I ordered from various merchants only to be disappointed by a chalky texture or by a bitter, artificial after-taste. Finally, by a stroke of luck, I came upon Maine Cottage Foods — purveyors of the very best chocolates and baked goods for diabetics. In addition to colorful, foiled-wrapped, chocolate teenies (6 teenies for an unbelievable 2 grams of carbs), they also have invented a line of baked goods made exclusively with almond flour and whey protein. The tiny, glazed brownies are a succulent revelation: deep chocolate flavor in bite-size portions for less than 4 grams of carb. Topping these fabulous morsels with no sugar/non-fat whipped topping and circling this confection with fresh, sweet raspberries will make the most ardent carb-counter feel happy to be alive.

Using the limits and structure I learned from Dr. Bernstein, I began to conceive of a cookbook which would create 16 meals, 4 for each season of the year. Each meal would feature a dessert and would total 20 grams or less of carb per person.

Inspired by Maine Cottage Foods and their inventions, I studied almond flour and its properties for baking. I learned how to make an almond flour torte, featuring dark chocolate "jewels" from Maine Cottage Foods. Then I learned how to make almond flour pancakes, moist and dense with flavor and rich in protein. These treats are featured in our cookbook.

No one was more supportive as I faced the challenge of dodging diabetes than Martha. As a physician, she understands very well the threat diabetes poses to the body. As a food lover, she appreciates the impact of a seriously restricted diet and understands how I dreaded it. Together, over the last three years, we tested my little discovery: *daVinci* syrups (sugar-free) poured over yogurt and made into sweet summer drinks (some with a splash of half-and-half). We talked about the growing incidence of prediabetes and diabetes in this country and around the world. We worried together about the impact on children as obesity sets in early, brought on by a high-sugar diet and an increasingly sedentary lifestyle. We worried about my health together which helped me decide to create a sustainable, livable and enjoyable food life at the same time that I worked to avoid diabetes.

Our cookbook, *Dodging Diabetes Deliciously: A Low-Carb Approach to Prediabetes*, is a true joint effort. Martha and I have discussed each menu in detail, making decisions about how best to "spend" our carb grams. I have shopped and cooked while Martha has done the consulting, the dining and the beautiful photography. We hope that our cookbook appeals to your eye as well as to your palate. The images here bear witness to what we have discovered. It is possible to create simple, easily prepared meals that are as delicious as they are healthful. Doing so has been a feast in itself. Serving these meals to family, friends and loved ones has been cause for celebration.

All 16 meals have been tested on my sensitive, carbohydrate-challenged metabolism, and I have shared the results with you. They have met the test of safe post-meal blood sugar levels as well as the standards of my easily bored and discerning palate.

We hope using this book will renew your optimism about your own health and about a way forward to share the joy of food with those you love.

Introduction

by Martha Snider, M.D.

My love of food also goes back a long way and has led to some conflicting messages. When I was growing up, visits to the doctor always ended the same way: a discussion about my weight, a diet that no kid would eat, a shot to prevent some awful disease, and a brightly colored lollipop.

Without looking, I knew that candy wasn't on the printed diet that the doctor had handed my mother.

Fast-forward a few decades. By this time, I had lost weight.

My friend, Connie, and I started working on a cookbook for people at risk of developing diabetes. While researching for the text, I came across and bought yet another book about diet and abnormal metabolism. The cover prominently displayed the name of a renowned medical institution.

In the nutrition section, one recipe after another contained the following ingredients: sugar, brown sugar, powdered sugar, cornstarch, honey. One recipe recommended adding sugar to asparagus.

I grew up in the deep South where love and food are synonymous, where meats *and* vegetables are deep fried and washed down by gallons of sweet tea. Even *we* don't add sugar to our vegetables.

Since the time of Connie's diagnosis with prediabetes, I have grappled with reconciling her experience — and the supporting experience and advise of physicians such as Richard Bernstein, Steve Parker and others — with conflicting recommendations published by organizations whose directives I had previously accepted without question. Prior to the past several years, I had assumed that standard dietary recommendations from qualified sources were effective if "taken to heart" and followed.

Although I might have known intuitively that someone with prediabetes would not metabolize bread or cereal or super-sweet fruit the same way a non-prediabetic would, I learned from Connie's blood glucose readings just *how* different and how *sensitive* prediabetic metabolism can be when it comes to carbs.

Now, when I read a publication intended specifically for prediabetics that encourages a diet with "plenty of fruits, vegetables and whole grains," I question whether this diet is right for all members of its intended audience.

Admittedly, it wasn't until the last few years that I have given much thought to the fact that not all fruits are created equal, nor all vegetables for that matter, or that grains — even whole, sprouted, fiber-rich ones (in regular serving sizes) — would not necessarily be healthy for everybody.

And, as chief taste tester for this cookbook, I can say that I have loved every bite of every meal my friend, the chef, has prepared, and I found them completely satisfying without unnecessary carbs and without any sugar added to the vegetables! One of Connie's objectives has been to create meals that are not merely tolerable for someone at high risk for developing diabetes, but meals that are appealing to anyone who enjoys food. In my view, she has succeeded.

Why do we care?

The concern about diabetes is dear to both our hearts. The disease shaves years off people's lives and interferes with the quality of those lives along the way.

I want to emphasize an important point. Looking from the outside, aware that diabetes and related disorders cause serious medical problems, the act of eating more and more of particularly unhealthy foods seems misguided. In many cases, however, that is not at all how it *feels*. Strong neuro-chemical and hormonal factors — those that have allowed our species to survive — drive eating behavior. One common hormonal abnormality causes people who have more-than-adequate fat stores and who have had plenty to eat to feel as if they are starving.[1]

Both the science *and* the politics surrounding the obesity and diabetes pandemic are fascinating. Suffice it to say, it wasn't just biology that lead to the current crisis.

A brief bit of dietary history: back in the 1980s, because of concern about the high

[1] See page 68.

incidence of heart disease and the belief that it was a direct result of high amounts of dietary fat, the American Medical Association, the Food and Drug Administration and others advised us to eat less fat. The food industry responded by removing fat from prepared foods and adding sugar and high fructose corn syrup in its place.

Researchers use the word "addictive" in reference to sugar and other fructose-rich sweeteners, in part, because these substances have been shown to activate the same chemicals in the brain that are affected by morphine and heroin. The food industry has capitalized on this biological vulnerability and, similar to the tactics used in the past by the tobacco industry (with Joe Camel), has marketed many of its products directly to children.

To whatever degree we have control over our eating behaviors or our food environment, some of us get motivated by thinking about the producers of carb-laden fast foods raking in huge profits while parents and their children develop diabetes.

The "diet food" industry makes billions too. I continually am amazed at how much sugar/refined carbohydrate is contained in so-called diet foods. The carbohydrate we eat causes insulin secretion, and insulin causes the body to store fat.

For people at risk for diabetes (which is quickly becoming almost all of us), the less refined carbohydrate we have, the better. For others (who can determine for themselves whether this applies), the less carbohydrate they eat period, the better. None of this is to say that either Connie or I advocate deprivation. In fact, we are totally anti-deprivation. We both absolutely love food and believe in getting the most pleasure from it that we can.

As we developed *Dodging Diabetes Deliciously*, my initial role was as a photographer, a taste tester, and a supportive friend. Now, as I have become involved in the writing, my intention is not to give advice — medical or otherwise.

There are scores of cookbooks available that *do* offer all kinds of advice. The trouble is that many of the most authoritative-sounding ones absolutely contradict one another. Each, no doubt, has validity and usefulness for some percentage of the population. Low-carb, wheat-free, and vegan are all healthy ways to eat — some better for the planet than others, some better for prediabetic metabolism than others.

The question is: which plan to follow?

The truth is that I'm chomping at the bit to give all kinds of advice. Instead, I will offer a few not-so-random sentences and suggestions:

- Anyone who is curious about the way his/her body handles a carbohydrate "load" — especially if that person has a family history of diabetes, carries extra weight around the middle, is over 40 years of age, or is a person of color — can obtain vitally important information by having a blood sugar test done. The more any of us knows about our own metabolism, the more empowered we are to decide what advice to follow.

- Become interested in food politics. Find out about food lobbies and the methods used to influence public policy. Support efforts to improve the food environment for the next generation.

- Exercise with a friend.

- Don't be fooled by false health claims regarding the benefits of processed, high-carb foods.

- Think of ways to celebrate birthdays (the gift of life) without traditional ice cream and cake.

- Get pleasure and comfort in lots of different ways.

- Try some of the dishes you find described and pictured on the following pages. See whether you are more satisfied, have fewer cravings, or have better numbers (if you check those). Become your own science experiment.

- If you don't want to experiment, that's fine also. Maybe you just like delicious-tasting food. If that's your thing, you are in for a big treat! May you be well, treat yourself well and enjoy.

Table of Contents

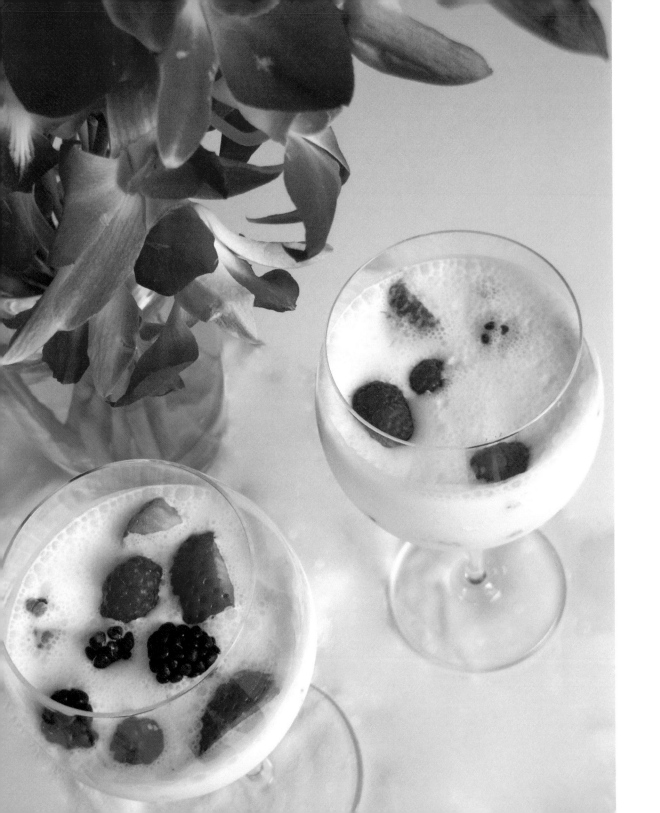

Spring

Spring Mother's Day Pancake Brunch

Ingredients *(for 2 servings)*:

⅔ cup Red Mill ground almond flour

2 tablespoons baking powder

2 eggs, beaten

¼ cup canola oil

Pinch of salt

8 drops *EZ-Sweetz* (liquid sucralose)

1 teaspoon almond extract

2 tablespoons butter

daVinci sugar-free syrup (available from netrition.com)

½ pint heavy whipping cream

1 pint raspberries

Make pancakes with almond flour, eggs, canola oil, *EZ-Sweetz*, vanilla extract and a pinch of salt and use your cast iron frying pan as a griddle. Melt butter in griddle to fry pancakes. Top pancakes with real whipped cream (very low-carb). Make a lovely coulis with raspberries swirled in the blender with *daVinci* sugar-free syrup. So easy, delicious and festive!

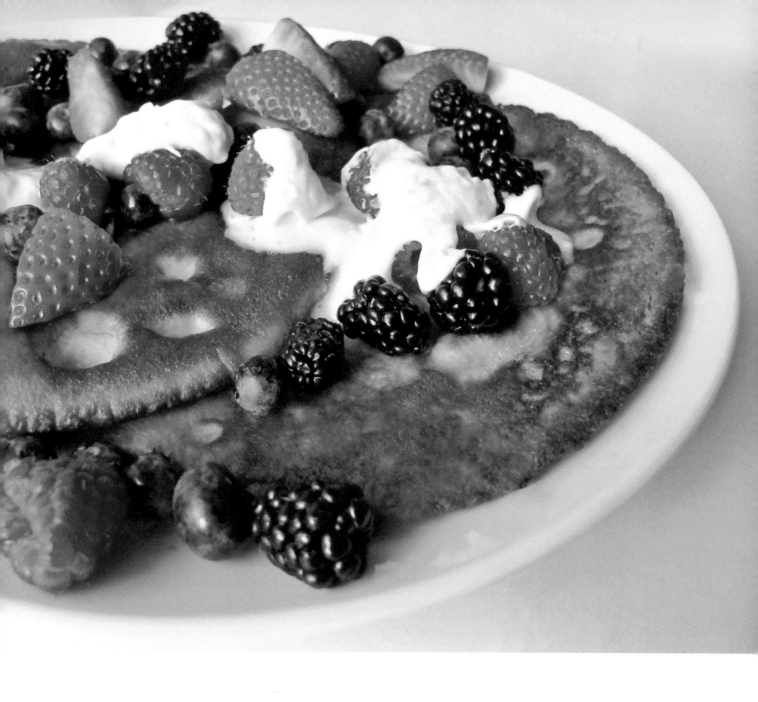

Spring Lamb

PRE-TEST: 100
POST-TEST: 112
CARBS: 14.5 grams
per serving

Ingredients *(for 2 servings)*:

2 pastured lamb chops (1.5 – 2 inches thick)

Kosher salt, pepper and ground rosemary

1 cup shaved Parmesan cheese

Salad: 4 cups salad greens including arugula, beet greens and fresh spring lettuces plus
½ cup cooked quinoa, ½ cup black beans, and 3 tablespoon sunflower seeds

Salad dressing: ½ cup virgin olive oil, 1 tablespoon *Bragg's Liquid Aminos,* and
4 tablespoons mixed red wine vinegar and balsamic vinegar

1 lb. steamed asparagus

For Dessert:

Small glazed chocolate brownies from Maine Cottage Foods

1 can non-fat/no sugar whipped cream from Whole Foods

1 pint strawberries

This meal would be fitting for Easter or Passover (although it is not kosher) or for a festive celebration of spring equinox.

First sear lamb chops in a cast iron pan and then roast them at 400° for a few minutes. Serve with steamed asparagus, a side salad and Parmesan crisps. To make crisps, simply place Parmesan on a baking dish in small dollops and bake for 10 minutes at 350°, checking a few times. These crisps are crunchy, salty and double as matzoh.

Our side salad is composed of fresh

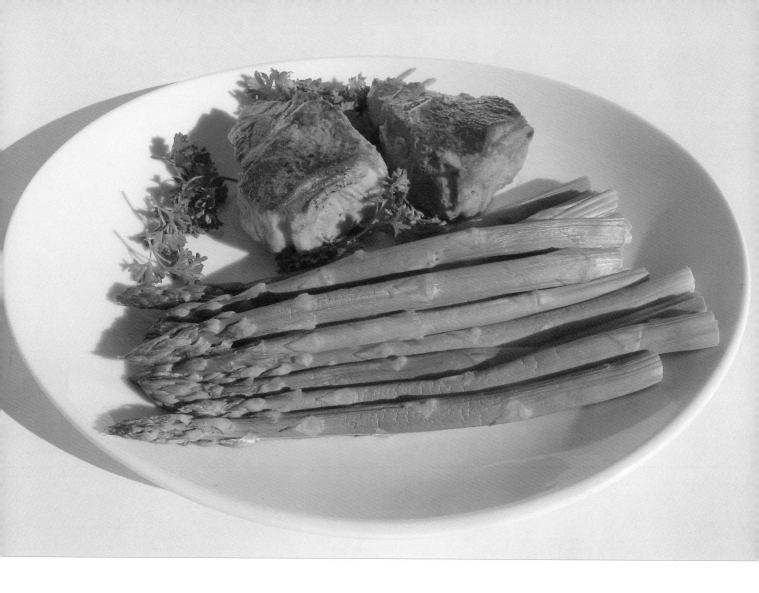

spring greens and quinoa, black soy beans and sunflower seeds with a simple vinaigrette dressing. For the dressing, use 2 parts olive oil to 1 part mixed balsamic/red wine vinegar and 1 tablespoon of *Bragg's Liquid Aminos* (a very low-sodium soy sauce available everywhere).

For dessert, serve fresh strawberries with non-fat whipped cream (no sugar/no carbs, available at Whole Foods) and a small chocolate brownie with a chocolate jewel on top of the whipped cream.

Spring Vegetarian Salad

PRE-TEST: 104
POST-TEST: 114
CARBS: 14.5 grams
per serving

Ingredients *(for 2 servings)*:

8 cups crispy local lettuces, spinach, arugula, green pepper and red cabbage

½ cup crumbled goat cheese

½ pint fresh raspberries

1 cup toasted walnuts (we use a cast iron skillet for toasting — watch them closely to avoid scorching)

Salad dressing: ½ cup olive oil, ¼ cup balsamic vinegar and 2 tablespoons *Bragg's Liquid Aminos*

1 pint fava bean hummus (available at Whole Foods — about half the carb count of regular hummus)

1 cup shaved Parmesan cheese for Parmesan crisps

For Dessert:

1 pint frozen raspberries

2 cups unsweetened almond/coconut milk

1 tablespoon almond extract

10 drops *EZ-Sweetz (liquid sucralose)*

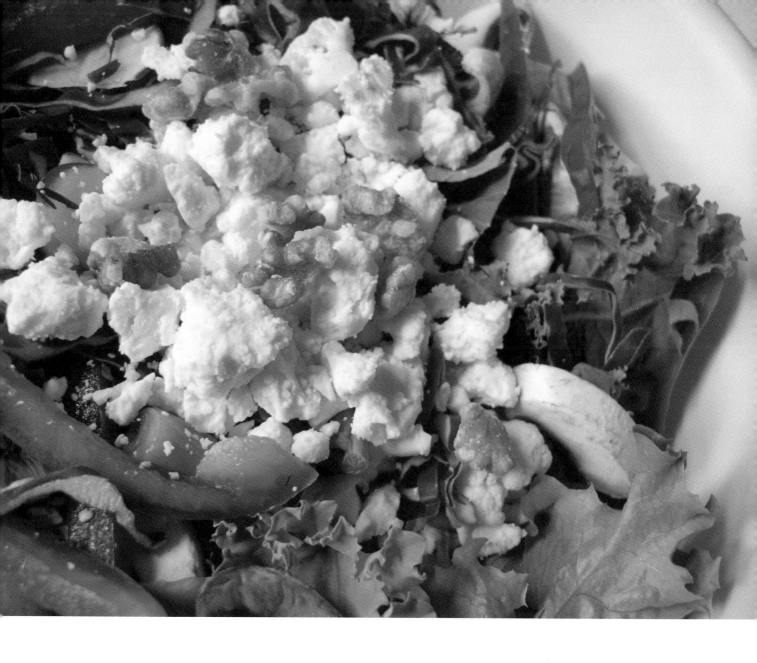

Every season brings fresh produce — organic, local and sustainable, grown in farms close by to where we live in Berkeley.

To create a salad bowl filled with this abundance, choose crispy local lettuce, spinach, arugula, crumbled goat cheese, toasted walnuts, and fresh local raspberries. Serve fava bean hummus on Parmesan crisps. These crisps couldn't be easier or more delicious. Pre-heat the oven to 350° and mound up some freshly grated Parmesan. In 5 minutes they have melted into a round "crackers" with irregular edges.

To round out this celebration of Spring, make one of our creamy, refreshing berry sorbets in the blender. Freeze the berries and add unsweetened almond/coconut milk (just 40 calories per full 8 oz. cup and 2 grams of carb). Add a few drops of our favorite *EZ-Sweetz* and about one tablespoon of organic almond extract.

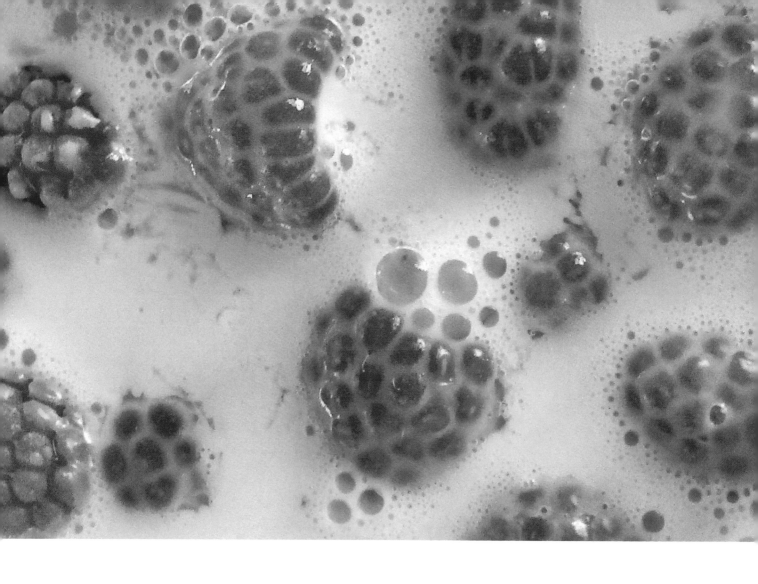

Spring Halibut

PRE-TEST: 101
POST-TEST: 120
CARBS: 15.5 grams
per serving

Ingredients *(for 2 servings)*:

1 lb. fresh halibut fillet

Cajun Dry Rub

1 cup dry white wine

1 cup prepared guacamole (Trader Joe's is excellent)

1 lemon

1 bunch kale, center rib removed

1 bulb garlic

1 ripe avocado

Salad: 3 cups fresh mixed greens including spinach, arugula and endive plus ½ cup toasted almonds, ½ cup canned chickpeas (garbanzos), ½ cup crumbled goat cheese

Salad Dressing: ½ cup olive oil, ¼ cup balsamic vinegar and 2 tablespoons *Bragg's Liquid Aminos*

For Dessert:

(all ingredients in blender)

1 cup low-fat ricotta

1 cup 2% *Fage* Greek yogurt

2 teaspoons almond extract

10 drops *EZ-Sweetz* (liquid sucralose)

¼ cup unsweetened almond milk

1 cup assorted berries for topping

Season the halibut with *Cajun Dry Rub*. Poach it with white wine in a pre-heated 375° oven for 20 minutes. Decorate with lemon wedges and guacamole. Serve braised kale sautéed quickly in hot olive oil with whole garlic cloves. For a mixed salad, assemble avocado (a wonderful source of omega 3), toasted almonds, and chickpeas over arugula, baby spinach, and

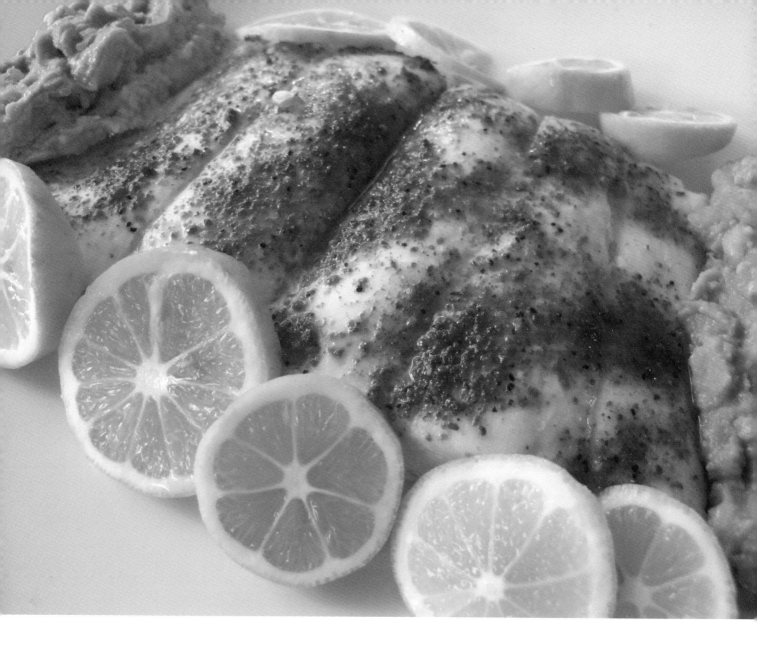

endive — tossed with a basic vinaigrette to which has been added 1 tablespoon of *Bragg's Liquid Aminos*.

For dessert, serve a special low-carb panna cotta: ricotta, yogurt and unsweetened almond milk blended with almond extract. Floating raspberries, blackberries, and blueberries finish this light pudding.

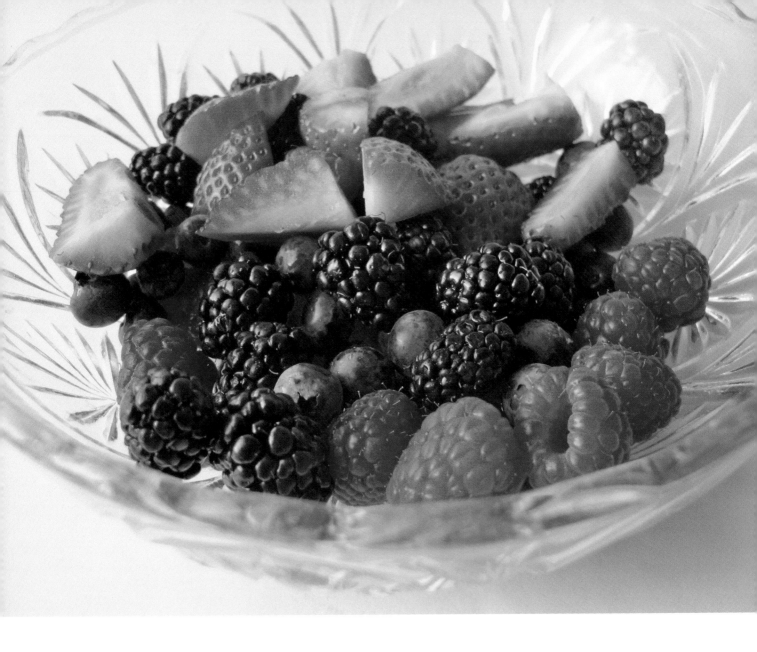

Summer

Summer Burger

PRE-TEST: 102
POST-TEST: 123
CARBS: 16.5 grams
per serving

Ingredients *(for 2 servings)*:

1 lb. pastured ground beef: half chuck and half rib eye

Sautéed vegetable medley: ½ lb. snap peas, 1 large onion, 1 each: red/yellow/orange bell pepper, 2 zucchini, and 1 lb. mixed mushrooms

1 garnet yam

Salt and pepper, to taste

For Dessert:

1 cup low-fat ricotta

1 cup 2% *Fage* Greek yogurt

½ cup chocolate "jewels" from Maine Cottage Foods

1 pint fresh raspberries

Summer sends out a siren call for burgers. Shape the ground beef into 4 patties. Brush both sides with oil and season. Sear the patties in a very hot, well-seasoned cast iron skillet. Finish them in a 400° oven for just a few minutes to achieve medium rareness.

Serve with a sautéed vegetable medley: onion, bell peppers, mushrooms, zucchini and snap peas. For this meal, add a few roasted yam chunks on the side both for color and a bit of sweetness.

Cut the yam into cubes, toss in olive oil and roast in a 400° oven for 45 minutes.

For this summer low-carb feast, compose a layered parfait of ricotta cheese, low-fat yogurt, unsweetened chocolate "jewels" and fresh raspberries. This dessert has just the right tangy sweetness.

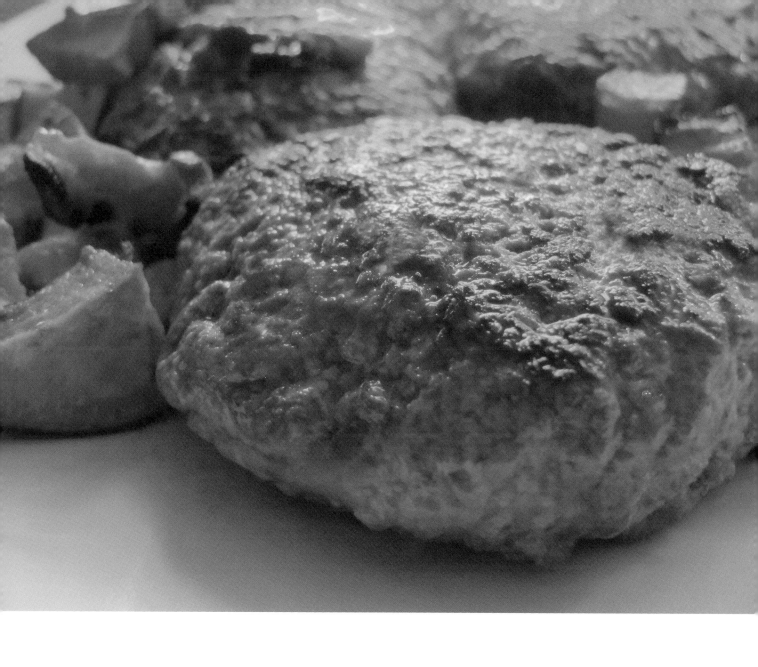

Summer Salmon

PRE-TEST: 105
POST-TEST: 117
CARBS: 17.5 grams
per serving

Ingredients *(for 2 servings)*:

2 2-inch thick wild salmon steaks

Just Cook N°19 Salmon Seasoning Blend (available online)

1 lemon

4 tablespoons olive oil for seasoning fish and cooking vegetables

1 lb. string beans (Blue Lake are best)

½ cup toasted slivered almonds

1 each: red, yellow and orange bell pepper, sautéed until browned

For Dessert:

1 pint frozen raspberries

2 cups unsweetened almond/coconut milk

10 drops *EZ-Sweetz* (liquid sucralose)

Season two thick salmon steaks with *N°19* seasoning and sear them at high heat in the cast iron skillet before finishing them in a 375° oven for about 6 minutes, testing for doneness. Serve the salmon with steamed local string beans garnished with toasted almonds and sautéed mixed peppers.

For dessert, serve a frozen blended berry sorbet.

Pour 1 pint of frozen raspberries and 2 cups of unsweetened almond milk into the blender, add a splash of vanilla extract and about 10 drops of *EZ-Sweetz*. The sorbet has a perfect creamy finish. Serve raspberry lemonade with this summer meal.

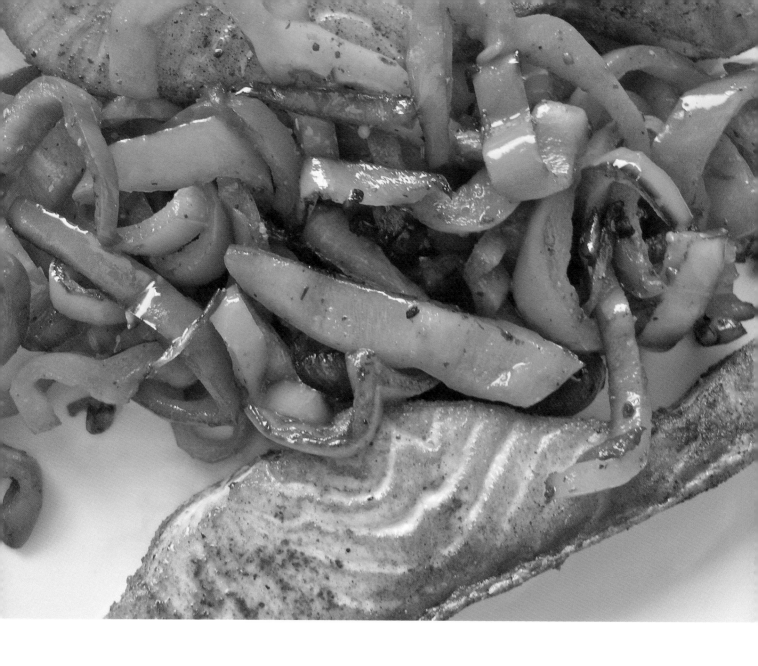

Summary Chicken

PRE-TEST: 110
POST-TEST: 122
CARBS: 16.5 grams
per serving

Ingredients *(for 2 servings)*:

4 boneless, skinless chicken thighs

2 tablespoons Thai Garlic Chili sauce (from Whole Foods)

1 lb. shiitake mushrooms

1 pint non-fat sour cream

½ cup Vermouth

1 bunch (or 1 lb.) asparagus spears

1 small cauliflower

½ cup shaved Parmesan cheese

4 tablespoons olive oil

1 tablespoon *Bragg's Liquid Aminos*

For Dessert:

2 brownies from Maine Cottage Foods

½ cup marscapone cheese

6 chocolate teenies (orange zest)
  from Maine Cottage Foods

Marinate the chicken thighs overnight in the Thai Garlic Chili sauce thinned with 2 tablespoons olive oil. Make the mushroom sauce, sautéing the shiitakes in 2 tablespoons olive oil. Add the Vermouth and let the mushrooms cook until they are soft and fragrant. It is best to add the sour cream at the end to prevent curdling.

Sear the marinated chicken thighs in a very hot cast iron skillet with 1 tablespoon of olive oil. Having set the oven to 400°, toss the cauliflower florets (separated into even-sized pieces) in another tablespoon of olive oil and an equal amount of *Bragg's Liquid Aminos*. Roast the cauliflower florets until they are browned (for about 20 minutes).

Lightly steam the asparagus spears and toss them with shaved Parmesan. After the cauliflower is roasted, finish the chicken thighs in a 350° oven for another 10 minutes. Serve the chicken covered with mushroom sauce, roasted cauliflower, and steamed asparagus topped with Parmesan.

The small glazed brownies are dressed with a generous dollop of creamy marscapone and finished with two foiled wrapped orange zest teenies for a welcome taste of chocolate at meal's end.

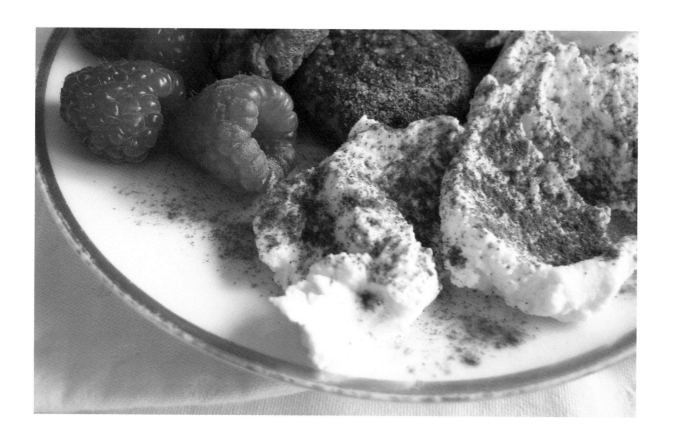

Summer Spinach Salad

PRE-TEST: 104
POST-TEST: 116
CARBS: 17.5 grms
per serving

Ingredients *(for 2 servings)*:

6 cups salad greens including kale, arugula, spinach, turnip greens, and lettuces

1 cup canned garbanzo beans (a higher carb legume so we limit the quantity)

1 ripe avocado

4 oz. crumbled goat cheese

4 oz. roasted cashews with no salt

1 each: red, yellow and orange bell pepper

¼ lb. cherry tomatoes

Salad dressing: 1 clove fresh garlic, ½ cup olive oil, ¼ cup Balsamic vinegar,
2 tablespoons *Bragg's Liquid Aminos*

For Dessert:

1 pint frozen strawberries

1½ cups unsweetened almond milk

1 tablespoon almond extract

10 drops *EZ-Sweetz* (liquid sucralose)

Mix the dressing and set it aside. Then oil a large wooden salad bowl and rub it with a clove of fresh garlic. Toss the mixed greens with ribbons of pepper before adding garbanzos, avocado, goat cheese, tomatoes and cashews. Finally, pour dressing over the salad just before serving.

For dessert, blend one pint of frozen strawberries and 1½ cups of unsweetened almond milk, adding 10 drops of *EZ-Sweetz* and a tablespoon of almond extract. It is best to serve this immediately in chilled goblets.

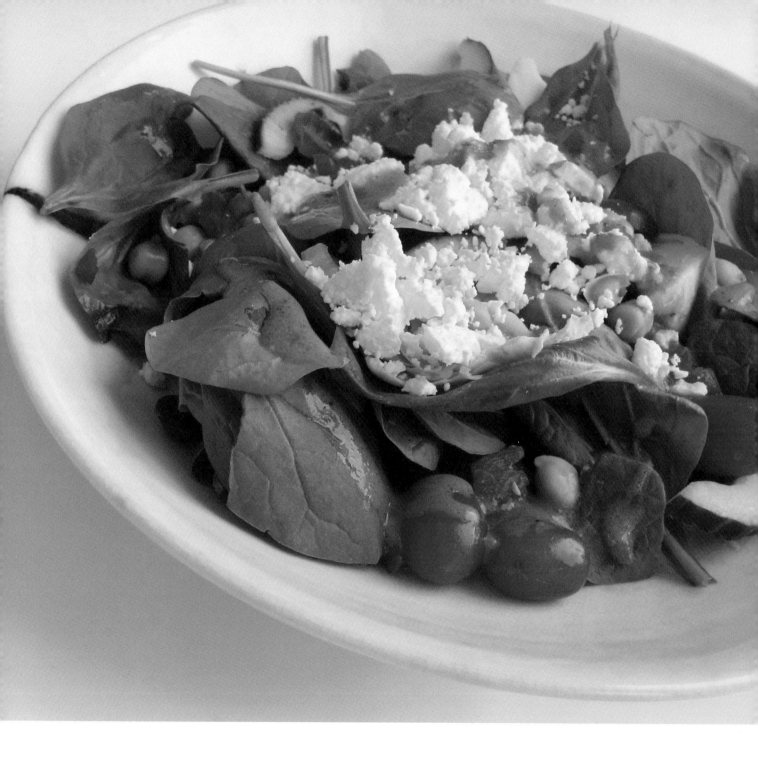

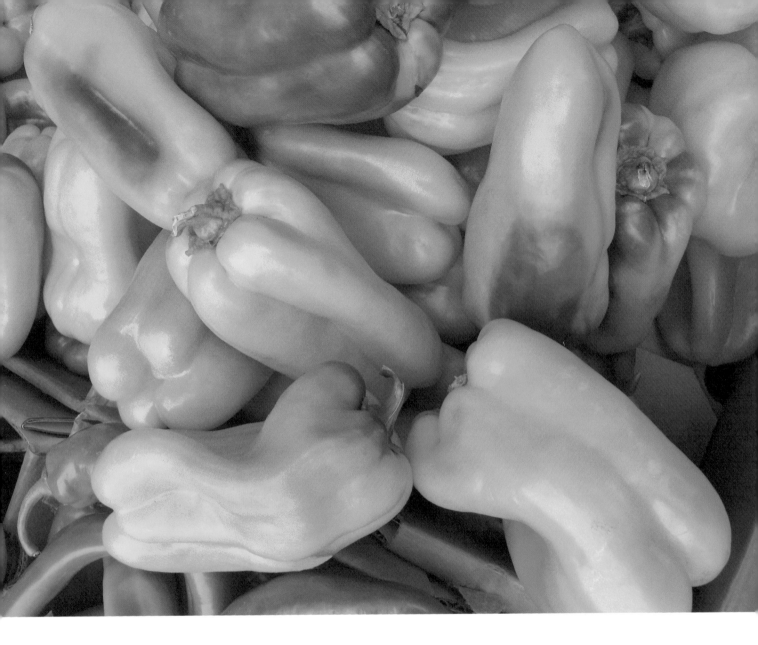

Fall

Thanksgiving

Ingredients *(for 2 servings)*:

4 Cornish hens

2 tablespoons Bell's poultry seasoning mixed with salt and pepper

Stuffing: 2 large onions, 1 bunch of celery, 1 cup toasted pecans, and 2 sliced firm apples (Gala or Granny Smith work best)

3 garnet yams (medium size) cut into cubes

1½ lbs. Brussels sprouts

2 jars peeled, steamed chestnuts

¼ lb. butter

1½ lb. string beans (Blue Lake are best)

1 lb. bag whole cranberries

1 large navel orange

1 lb. mushrooms

For Dessert:

EZ-Sweetz

16 oz. reduced fat Philadelphia cream cheese

1 can mashed organic pumpkin (mixed with two beaten eggs)

Dash of salt and two dashes of vanilla

1 tablespoon each: nutmeg, ginger and/or pumpkin pie spice

1 can non-fat/no sugar whipped cream

For a special holiday meal, serve tender Cornish game hens (with a traditional sage seasoning) accompanied by roasted yam, Brussels sprouts, chestnuts and string beans with mushrooms. First, wash, dry, season and roast the hens in a pre-heated 375° oven for 1 hour and 15 minutes. While the hens are roasting, combine the stuffing ingredients. Sauté in melted butter and bake separately in 375° oven for 1 hour. Cut the yams into cubes and roast in 400° oven for 30 minutes. Steam the Brussels sprouts briefly before sautéing in butter together with the chestnuts. Steam stringbeans separately and sauté quickly with mushrooms. Of course, cranberry sauce is *de rigueur*. For a tangy, citrusy sauce, combine organic

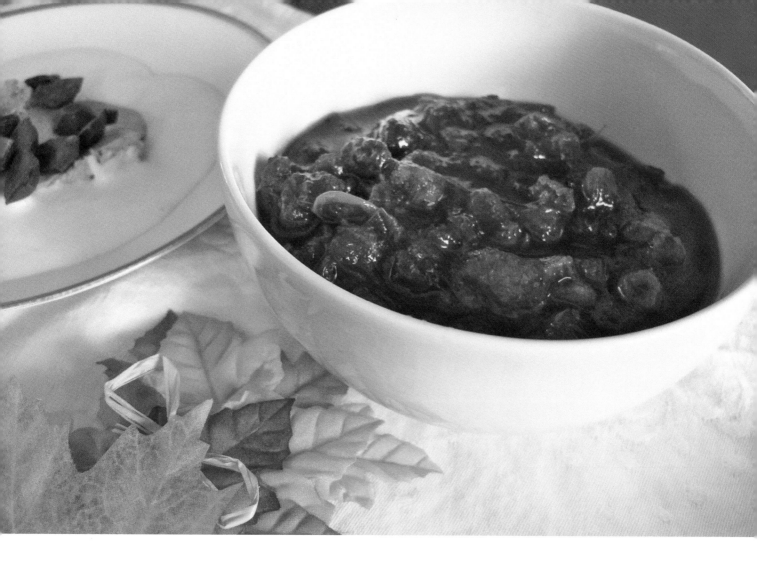

cranberries with a cut up orange and several drops of *EZ-Sweetz*.

Dessert is the *pièce de résistance* of this special meal. Staying close to the traditions of the holiday, create a pumpkin mousse. Use Philadelphia cream cheese, spices, canned pumpkin, *EZ-Sweetz,* and vanilla extract. Enjoy this pumpkin treat and never miss the crust.

For the mousse, combine all ingredients and mix by hand. Bake in 350° oven for 45 minutes. Test with a toothpick for desired doneness. Serve with not-fat/no sugar whipped cream.

Fall Duck

PRE-TEST: 95
POST-TEST: 116
CARBS: 18.5 grams
per serving

Ingredients *(for 2 servings)*:

2 large boned duck breasts

1 half-bottle Port wine

1 jar sugar-free apricot preserves (*Al 'n Jok* from netrition.com)

½ cup balsamic vinegar

1 lb. string beans (Blue Lake are best)

1 onion

1 each: red, yellow, orange bell pepper

Salad: 1 English cucumber, 1 ripe avocado, ½ cup toasted walnuts, ½ cup feta cheese, 10 radishes, 1 large endive

Salad dressing: ½ cup olive oil, ¼ cup balsamic vinegar, 1 tablespoon *Bragg's Liquid Aminos*

For Dessert:

2 glazed brownies from Maine Cottage Foods

1 cup non-fat/no sugar whipped cream (from Whole Foods)

Make the glaze for the duck breast first by reducing the Port, mixed with ½ cup balsamic vinegar and 3 tablespoons of non-sugar apricot preserves, until this mixture becomes a syrup. Set the syrup aside to serve separately and drizzle over the duck breasts.

After preheating the oven to 375°, season the duck breasts with salt and pepper and roast them for ½ hour before testing for doneness. They should be pink at the center. A meat thermometer registers 165° when the duck is finished cooking.

While the duck is roasting, slowly

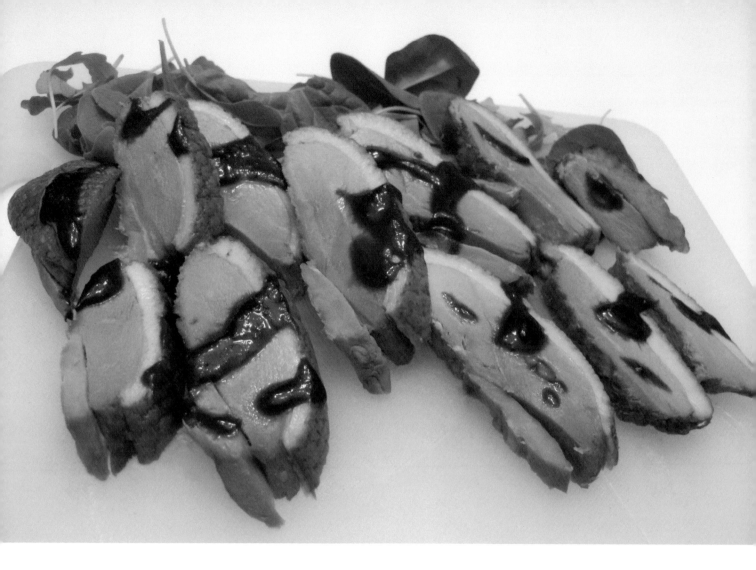

caramelize the onion in olive oil over low heat. When the onion is soft and brown, toss in the thinly sliced peppers and sauté them until they are softened and browned.

The salad we use to accompany the duck has no lettuce. Instead, it relies on cucumber, endive, radishes, and avocado, mixed together with toasted walnuts and feta cheese. Dress the salad right in the bowl, tossing it with olive oil, balsamic vinegar and a splash of *Bragg's Liquid Aminos*.

For dessert, serve a glazed brownie sitting on a bed of non-fat/no sugar whipped cream.

Fall Pork Loin

Ingredients *(for 2 servings)*:

3-lb. pork loin

Cajun Dry Rub (available online)

2 Japanese eggplants

2 tablespoons Thai Chili Garlic sauce (it has a bit of sugar)

1 large sweet onion

1 large red pepper

2 small apples (Honey Crisp are best)

1 stick butter

1 tablespoon cinnamon

For Dessert:

2 ricotta Baci from *Maine Cottage Foods*

1 pint fresh raspberries

Preheat oven to 375° and let loin roast come to room temperature. Season the pork loin with kosher salt, pepper and *Cajun Dry Rub* (a medium spicy, paprika based rub). Roast until the meat thermometer registers 180°. Test the roast using a sharp knife. We like our pork just the slightest bit pink but tastes vary.

Apples are a traditional accompaniment to pork loin. We bake ours alongside the meat in a separate Pyrex baking dish. It is important to slice these crisp apples evenly and lay them in one layer to bake. Dotted with butter and sprinkled with cinnamon, they add a sweet touch to the pork loin.

Season the evenly sliced Japanese eggplant with a thin layer of Chili Garlic sauce. Sauté one sweet onion and red pepper. Add the eggplant last and toss everything together before serving.

The pork loin is served in thin slices, covered with baked apples.

For dessert, assemble two Baci (the Italian word for "kisses") per plate and serve them with a mound of fresh ricotta sprinkled with cinnamon.

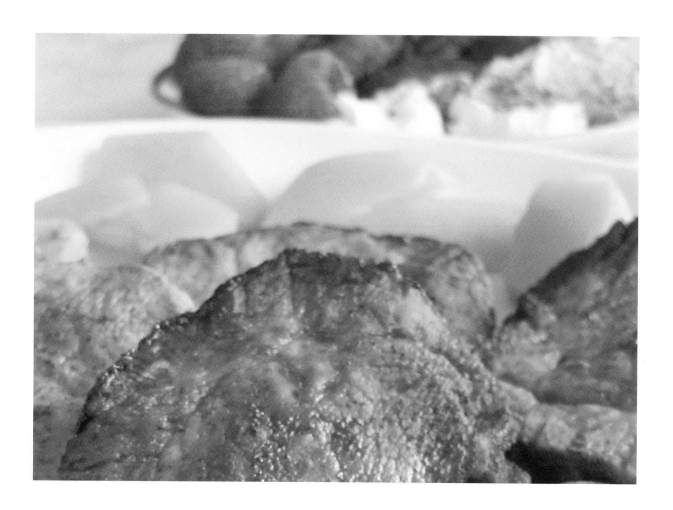

Fall Baked Tofu

PRE-TEST: 104
POST-TEST: 119
CARBS: 18.5 grms
per serving

Ingredients *(for 2 servings)*:

1 lb. firm frozen tofu, defrosted

½ pint fresh pesto sauce

2 tablespoons toasted sesame oil

1 tablespoon *Bragg's Liquid Aminos*

1 tablespoon Thai Chili Garlic sauce

1 head cauliflower, broken into
  equal-sized florets

1 lb. snap peas

2 cloves garlic

For Dessert:

¾ cup ground almond meal from *Red Mill*

2 eggs beaten

Pinch of salt

⅓ cup canola oil

1 rounded tablespoon baking powder

1 tablespoon almond extract

3 tablespoons slivered almonds

8 drops *EZ-Sweetz*

¼ cup chocolate "jewels" from
  Maine Cottage Foods

1 can non-fat/no sugar whipped cream

Slice the squeezed and rinsed defrosted tofu into equal-sized pieces. Mix together the sesame oil, Thai Garlic Chili sauce and *Bragg's Liquid Amino*s and marinate these slices for an hour.

Preheat the oven to 400°, coat the cauliflower florets with olive oil and *Bragg's* as evenly as possible. Then roast the florets for 30 minutes and set aside.

Layer the marinated tofu slices in an oiled baking dish and bake them for 20 minutes until golden brown. While the tofu slices bake, stir-fry snap peas in a hot skillet with 1 tablespoon of olive oil.

Assemble the baked tofu slices, roasted cauliflower and quick stir-fried snap peas on a platter and serve with pesto sauce on the side.

For the almond cupcakes, combine dry ingredients separately from wet ingredients and then mix together. Pour mixture into oiled cupcake molds. Bake in preheated 350° oven for 20 minutes. Set out to cool. Serve cupcakes on a bed of whipped cream, topped with "jewels".

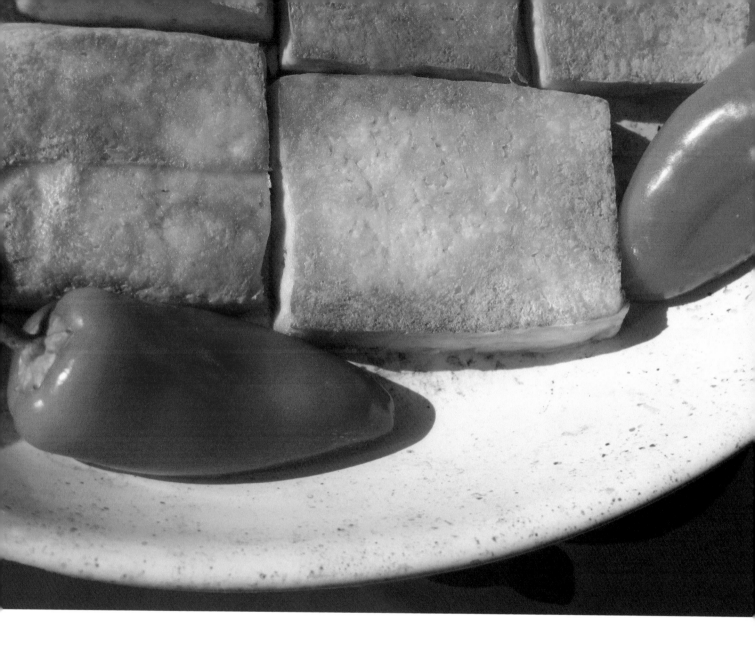

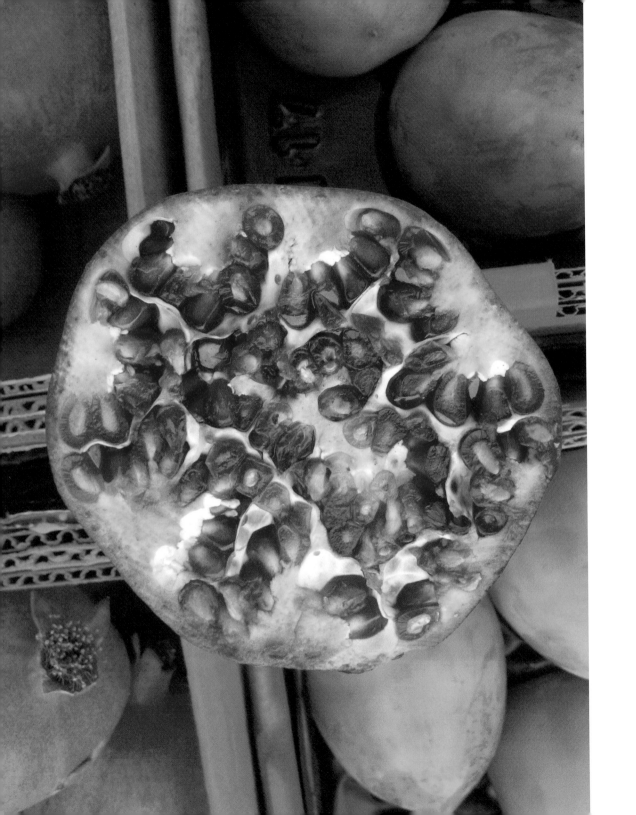

Winter

Christmas/Chanukah

PRE-TEST: 105
POST-TEST: 126
CARBS: 19.5 grms
per serving

Ingredients *(for 2 servings)* :

3 ribs of Prime Standing Rib Roast

Salt and pepper, to taste

1 spaghetti squash

2 lbs. fresh string beans (Blue Lake are best)

1 lb. button mushrooms

Salad: 1 cup each endive, maché, radicchio, and arugula lettuces; plus
½ cup each: toasted pecans, pomegranate seeds, Gorgonzola cheese (crumbled)

Salad dressing: ½ cup olive oil, 2 tablespoons *Bragg's Liquid Aminos*, 4 tablespoons
mixed red wine/balsamic vinegar

For Dessert:

1 cup ground almond flour
(Red Mill is best)

½ cup canola oil

2 tablespoons baking powder

2 eggs, beaten

Pinch of salt

1 tablespoon almond extract

10 drops *EZ-Sweetz*

For Topping:

1 pint fresh raspberries

½ cup ricotta

¼ cup *daVinci* no sugar raspberry syrup

Pomegranate seeds lend holiday red to this feast. Start the meal with a crunchy salad: arugula, endive, pomegranate seeds, slices of orange, Stilton cheese, toasted pecans, and vinaigrette. Then follow with a standing rib roast centerpiece entrée — accompanied by spaghetti squash with pecans and string beans with mushrooms as side dishes.

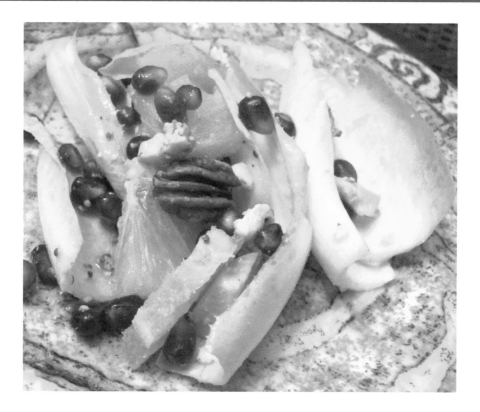

Pre-heat oven to 400°. Bring the meat to room temperature. Season with sea salt and ground pepper. Heat cast iron skillet until a droplet of water sizzles. Sear meat on both sides until brown. Place cast iron skillet in heated oven and roast meat until desired doneness. Check frequently with a sharp knife.

Roast spaghetti squash in a preheated 425° oven a day in advance. Then cut open, seed and mash with *Earth Balance,* salt and pepper. The button mushrooms are tossed with steamed string beans in 2 tablespoons

Earth Balance.

For the cake, combine dry and wet ingredients separately and then mix together. Oil the baking dish and bake for just 20 minutes in a 350° oven and allow the cake to sit in the oven for another 10 minutes with the oven door slightly ajar.

Decorate the almond flour torte with chocolate "jewels" from *Maine Cottage Foods* and drizzle blended raspberry sauce, mixed with ricotta, over the cake. Enjoy a glass of California Zinfandel with this special meal.

Winter Valentine Frittata

PRE-TEST: 94
POST-TEST: 112
CARBS: 12.0 grams
per serving

Ingredients *(for 2 servings)*:

4 eggs

1 lb. spinach

1 lb. mixed mushrooms (including shiitake, if available)

4 leeks

¾ cup mixed shaved Parmesan and Romano cheeses

½ cup milk

For Dessert:

Glazed brownies from *Maine Cottage Foods*

1 pint raspberries

1 pint non-fat/no sugar whipped cream

6 drops *EZ-Sweetz*

Vanilla extract

The spinach, mushrooms, and leeks are first gently sautéed in butter. Beat 4 eggs together with ½ cup milk and about ½ cup grated cheese. Add the sautéed vegetables to the beaten eggs and cheese. Gently cook the frittata in the cast iron skillet. Add the remaining cheese and brown it under the broiler for 3 minutes.

For dessert, serve the brownies with fresh raspberries and real whipped cream, sweetened with EZ-Sweetz and a few drops of vanilla extract.

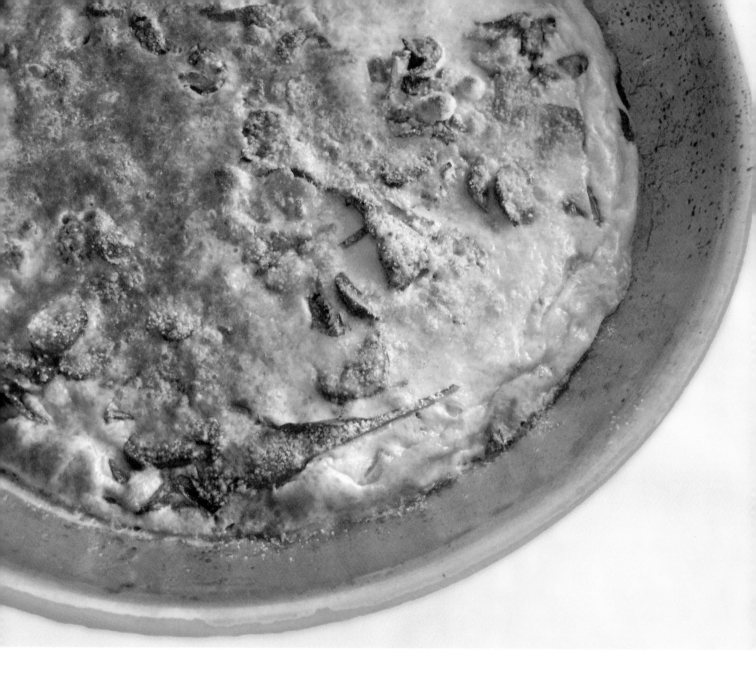

Winter Shrimp Stir-Fry

PRE-TEST: 87
POST-TEST: 110
CARBS: 18.5 grms
per serving

Ingredients *(for 2 servings)*:

1 lb. shelled and deveined medium-sized shrimp

3 tablespoons Thai Chili Garlic sauce

3 tablespoons olive oil

1 medium garnet yam

1 large sweet onion

1 each: red, yellow, and orange bell pepper

For Dessert:

2 6-oz. cups of *Fage* 2% Greek yogurt

1 bag frozen cranberries

1 small navel orange

10 drops *EZ-Sweetz*

Roast cubed garnet yam first in a preheated 400° oven for about 40 minutes and then set it aside.

Marinate the shrimp in the Thai Chili Garlic sauce for two hours before sautéing them in hot olive oil over high heat. Set the shrimp aside in a bowl. Caramelize the onion slowly in the same pan, adding another tablespoon of olive oil. When the onion is brown and soft, add the sliced bell peppers, turn up the heat and stir-fry them until brown and glistening. Finally, add the shrimp to the vegetables and pour the reduced glaze over both.

For dessert, make a cranberry sauce using the frozen berries, one navel orange cut into slices and 10 drops of *EZ-Sweetz*. First bring the berries and orange to a boil; then reduce the heat and let the fruit simmer until it is soft and fragrant. After the cranberry sauce cools, serve it over yogurt.

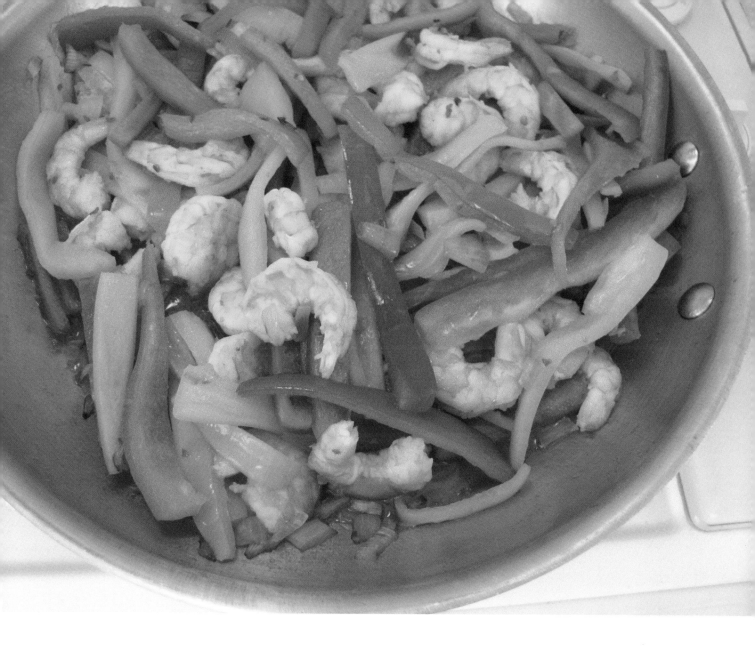

Winter Chicken Chili

PRE-TEST: 94
POST-TEST: 122
CARBS: 17.5 grams
per serving

Ingredients *(for 2 servings)*:

2 packaged boxes of Homestyle chicken chili (from netrition.com)

1 ripe chopped avocado

½ cup shredded mozzarella

1 each: red, yellow, and orange bell pepper

1 lb. stemmed string beans

1 lb. assorted mushrooms

3 tablespoons olive oil and kosher salt
  for vegetable sauté

For Dessert:

1 cup part-skim fresh ricotta

1 cup unsweetened almond milk

1 teaspoon almond extract

10 drops *EZ-Sweetz*

1 ripe Fuyu persimmon, thinly sliced

This fragrant, well-seasoned chili (made with low-carb black soy beans) goes well with mixed sautéed vegetables: string beans, peppers, onions, and a medley of seasonal mushrooms. Order packaged low-carb chicken chili. Serve it with side dishes of chopped avocado and grated mozzarella cheese. For a special dessert, thin ricotta cheese with ½ cup of half and half and add 1 teaspoon almond extract and a few drops of *EZ-Sweetz*. Pour into bowls and freeze for 10 minutes. Dress the frozen almond mousse with slices of fresh persimmon which really pop in Martha's wonderful photograph on the front cover.

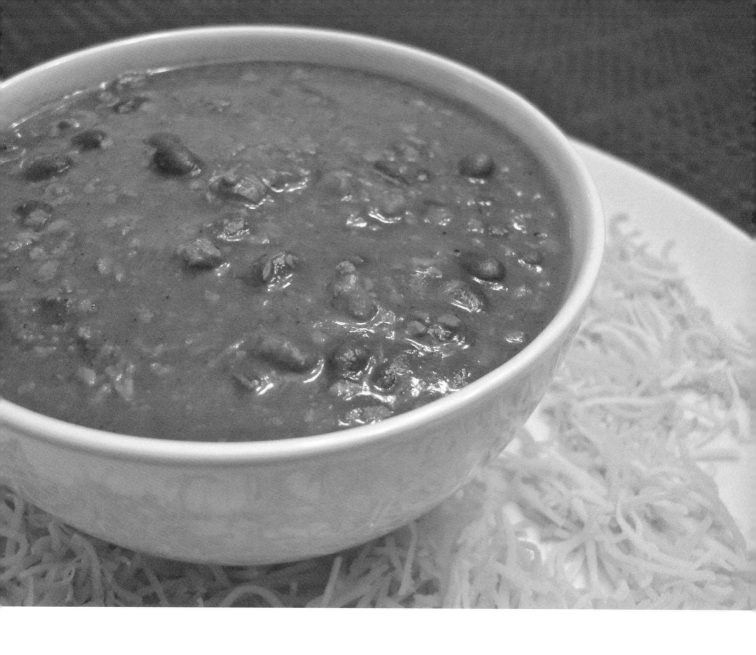

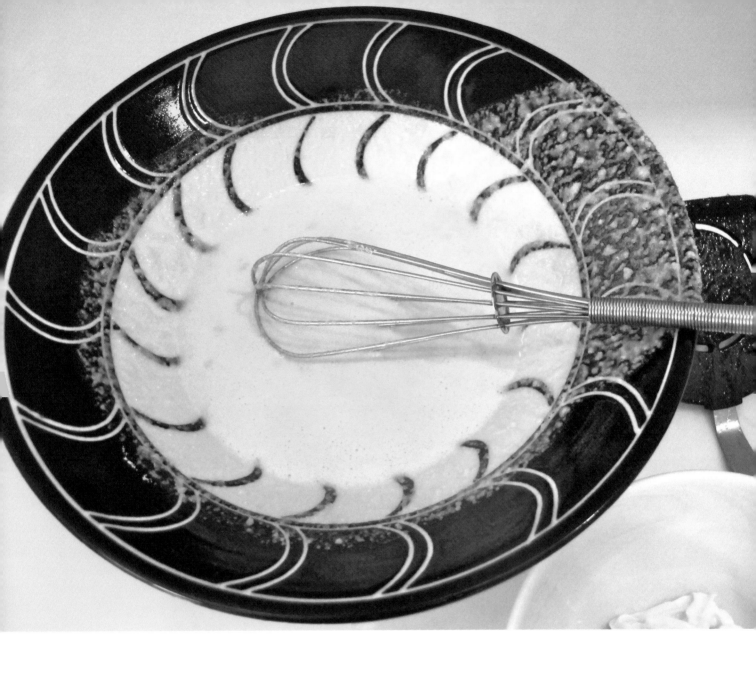

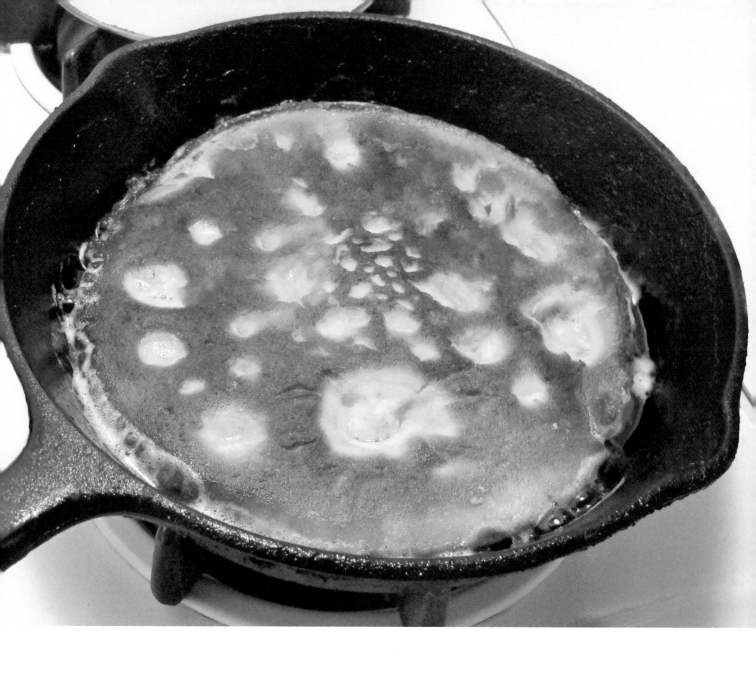

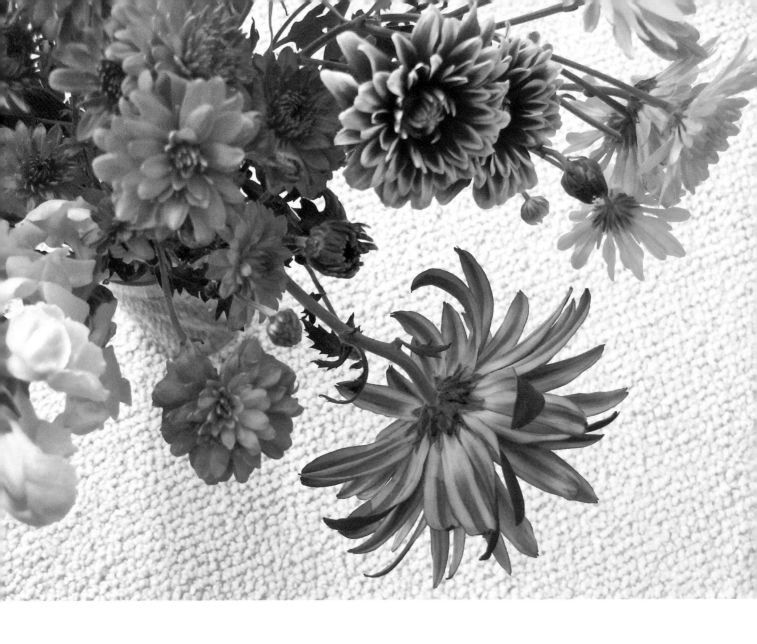

APPENDICES

ABOUT THE PHOTOGRAPHS

When I arrive at Connie's to take pictures of dinner, I am greeted with the aroma of sautéed mushrooms, yummy chili, or whatever other healthy low-carb offering she has prepared. The fragrances are what I notice first, and, of course, the light.

The plan is to photograph the food in natural light, before it cools. These won't be studio shots of inedible concoctions that look pretty but aren't intended to be eaten — such as pancakes drizzled with what looks like syrup, but is glue. Nope. This is real food.

For each shoot, not only are there edibles to please the eyes, but flowers as well. Lilies. Roses. Sweet peas — the floral kind.

For many of us foodies the end of a meal brings a sense of loss. Savoring the photographs hours and days later allows the pleasure to continue.

One of the themes of the photographs in *Dodging Diabetes Deliciously* is the "found mandala." Whether the rounded shape of the food — slices of lemons, brightly wrapped "teenies" from Maine Cottage Foods or the curve of a serving dish or pan — all suggest containment, and, in this context, awakening via the senses.

— M.S.

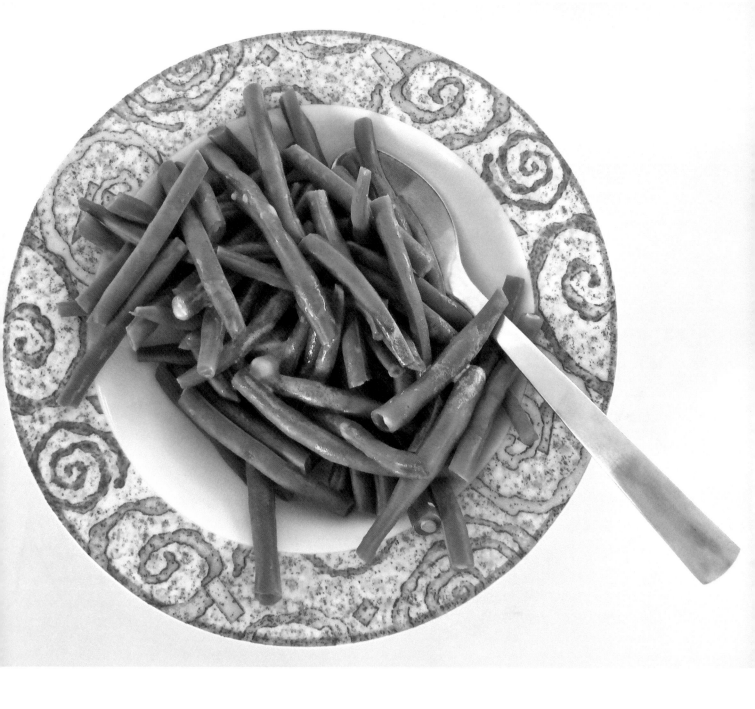

DEFINITIONS

The term *prediabetes* sounds as though it is a condition that comes before diabetes. It is true that a significant number of people with prediabetes do progress to a diagnosis of diabetes within three to five years, but not everyone does. Prediabetes is reversible.

A normal fasting blood sugar level is less than 100 mg/dl. A normal A1C level (which reflects average blood sugar values over the previous two to three months) is less than 5.7%.

Prediabetes is diagnosed if the A1C is 5.7 to 6.4 or if the fasting blood sugar tested on two separate occasions is between 100 and 125. Full-blown diabetes is diagnosed when A1C is 6.5 or greater or two fasting blood sugars are equal to or greater than 126.

By recent estimates from The Centers for Disease Control and Prevention, at least 25% of adult Americans (more than 60 million people) have prediabetes. And, according to multiple sources, fewer than 10% (probably significantly fewer) of the people who have prediabetes know that they have it!

Blood sugars of 140 or greater two hours after a meal have been shown to be associated with nerve damage and a sensation of "pins and needles" in the extremities. These symptoms were present in people who had prediabetes and didn't know that they had it. For some prediabetics, eating the amount of carbohydrate in *standard* diets recommended for their condition would push their after-a-meal blood sugars into the greater than 140 range.

There are several ways to reduce the risk of having prediabetes progress to diabetes. One is losing weight. Losing 14 to 20 pounds for someone who weights 200 pounds can be enough to reverse prediabetes. Moderate exercise several times a week also helps in preventing the progression of prediabetes to diabetes. Limiting or eliminating sugar whenever and however possible is a superb preventive strategy.

Type 1 diabetes, formerly referred to as juvenile diabetes or insulin dependent diabetes, is an autoimmune disease in which the insulin-producing cells in the pancreas are destroyed. The disease is treated by the administration of insulin.

Type 2 diabetes, previously called adult-onset diabetes, is the most prevalent form of diabetes and can occur in both adults and children.

Type 2 diabetes is associated with insulin

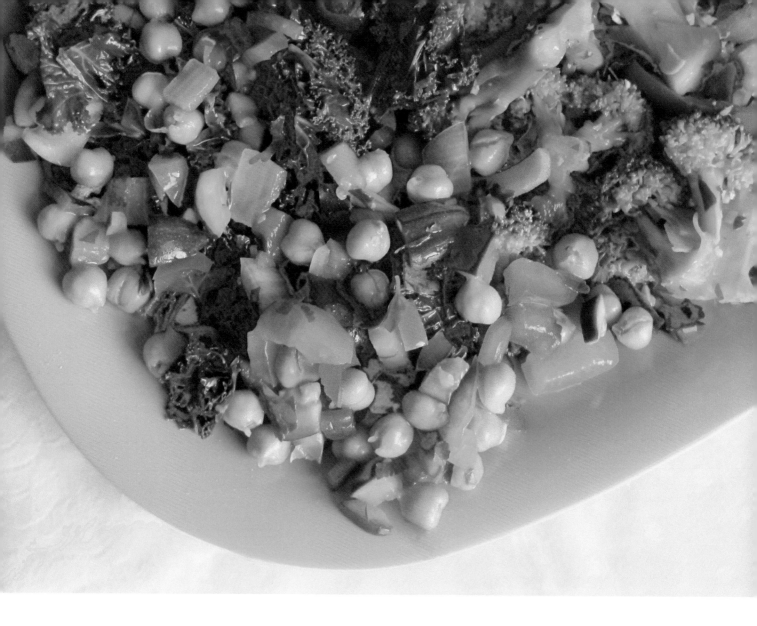

resistance, which results when the cells no longer respond to insulin properly. The condition is often, but not always, associated with being overweight. Initially the pancreas makes extra insulin in response to high blood sugar levels. Over time it isn't able to keep up with the demand and blood glucose levels rise. When prediabetes progresses to diabetes, it is type 2 diabetes that has developed.

Leptin is a hormone produced primarily by fat tissue. Leptin lets us know when we've had enough food and can stop eating. If the message doesn't get through, (in a condition known as leptin resistance), we keep on eating. As far as the person with leptin resistance is concerned, despite having eaten plenty of food and having adequate or more than adequate fat stores, it is as though they are starving. It feels wrong to *stop* eating.

If a person is starving, the fear of a heart attack or stroke or any other complication that might happen down the road doesn't mean much. It just doesn't come up.

In addition to influencing food intake, leptin also regulates energy expenditures. When a person's biology is sending a message of starvation, not only do they try to ingest as much food as possible (in the midst of what feels like a famine, who knows when the next food will be available?), the person also does everything they can to conserve energy. Movement is kept at a minimum. To get up and get moving feels wrong.

Leptin deficiency is very rare. Leptin resistance is much more common. The condition is linked to obesity.

WEIGHT LOSS AND THE TIMING OF MEALS

The periodical *Nutrition Action*[1] recently carried an article describing an Israeli study[2] about weight loss as it related to the timing of meals. Subjects in one group were instructed to eat the bulk of their calories at breakfast. Those in another were counseled to eat most of their daily caloric allotment at dinner. The number of calories for each group was the same. All were on a plan intended to help them lose weight. The results were not a surprise. Eating most of ones calories earlier in the day was associated with more weight loss, presumably because there was more time to expend the energy that was taken in.

[1] September 2013 issue.
[2] Published in *Obesity* 203.Doi:10.1002/Oby.20460.

LOSING WEIGHT AND KEEPING IT OFF

Years ago I met a woman named Helen who mentioned off-handedly that she had recently lost 60 pounds. I'm sure I looked interested. With very little prompting, Helen explained what she had done to lose weight.

The basics were pretty simple. The recommended allotment of food for a woman of my height (average) and activity level (a notch or two less than moderate) who wanted to lose weight[1] was the following:

  3 to 4 ounces of protein per meal
  2 to 3 cups of veggies for 2 meals per
      day (as a salad and/or cooked)
  1 serving of carbohydrate per meal
  2 servings of dairy per day
  2 pieces of fruit per day

Helen was explicit about what constituted a serving of carbohydrate: one slice of whole grain toast or ½ cup of cereal for breakfast, ½ cup of rice or a small potato or a small piece of bread at lunch and dinner.[2]

The fat component was specific too: a teaspoon of butter or oil at breakfast and one tablespoon of oil at the other two meals. Mixed with vinegar and a little mustard, that tablespoon of oil could become a dressing for a giant salad.

As I listened, I thought I might try what she was describing, at least temporarily. Some of the limitations seemed tolerable, but I was not willing to drag around feeling deprived all day. I needed at least one thing I could eat as much of as I wanted. Since there seemed to be more leeway with the vegetables, I decided to go *ad lib* on those. (Not exciting, but there was no *Dodging Diabetes Deliciously* back then.) With my one modification of all-you-can-eat vegetables, I decided to see if I could do what Helen said had worked for her.

Here's the surprise: I was less hungry eating limited portions of carbohydrates and fats than when I was eating a lot *more* food — far larger meals plus snacks off and on all day. What worked, as far as I can tell, was that I was getting enough protein, limiting my carbohydrate intake and not eating snacks. When I did have carbs of any kind — whether in milk, fruit, grains or starchy vegetables, I had protein at the same time.

Prior to this time, when I was eating an ordinary-American-diet amount of carbohydrate, I was hungry almost all the time. In retrospect, the high-carbohydrate snacks I was eating were likely jerking my blood sugar and insulin levels around. Following the plan that Helen described allowed me to lose weight at a rate of about 10 pounds per month. When I got to goal weight, I doubled — but still limited — the carbs. In addition to feeling less hungry, I had more energy.

Having been 50 or more pounds overweight in the past, nothing I had ever tried before worked as well or as sustainably for losing weight and keeping it off as limiting carbohydrates. It's now been 26 years.

With a little tweaking, keeping track of *grams* of protein instead of ounces, aiming for 20 grams of protein per meal, the plan is the same. As a point of reference, a three-ounce serving of chicken or fish has about 18 grams of protein, 8 ounces of milk (cow or soy) has 8 grams. Roasted soybeans with 12 grams per *quarter cup* are a great way to add protein to a meal, especially when there is not a lot of time to shop and prepare. Legumes are a great source of protein and a personal favorite, but they do have carbohydrates. A serving of beans would replace a serving of carbs.

The difference between the plan described above and the meals and recipes recommended for diabetes prevention in run-of-the-mill cookbooks is that the plan Helen described to me does not include refined carbohydrates in the form of sugar, "evaporated cane juice," high-fructose corn syrup, honey, or molasses as a major ingredient. If sugar is one of the first four ingredients on a label or one of the top four ingredients by weight in a recipe, I skip it. That's not to say that I do this perfectly, but for the most part I do.

Maybe giving up sugar was easier for me than it would have been for another person. Maybe I was not addicted. My hunch is that my hunger feedback loop was impaired, but not totally so.

Even though following this plan was easier than I expected when I first heard it, (I wasn't sure I could make it from lunch to dinner on Day 1), eating low-carb definitely presents some challenges. It goes against social norms. To be able to stick with it requires support.

Of all the people I know who have lost a hundred or more pounds and kept it off (I know several), all avoid sugar. Besides, sugar sets up cravings. Life is hard enough without feeling hungry all the time.

No recipe in *Dodging Diabetes Deliciously* has sugar as an ingredient.

---

[1] The author of this segment has normal blood glucose levels. The plan described has been shown to be effective for weight loss.

[2] For people with extremely carbohydrate-sensitive metabolism even ¼ cup of brown rice, a piece of fruit and a serving of dairy all in the same meal can cause a significant blood sugar spike.

STRESS EATING

Several years ago, at a medical meeting, I heard a presentation by a researcher who was studying the effects of stress hormones on sugar intake.

Experiments had been performed using mice. The study involved putting the test animals under stressful conditions and measuring their levels of cortisol and other stress hormones as well as observing the animals' behavior following the stress.

Being prey, mice respond to exposure, (being placed in the open on a raised platform), with an outpouring of cortisol. When offered various concentrations of sugar water to drink after this ordeal, the mice that had been left out in the open chose the highest concentration of sugar available. Mice in a control group, that had been left with the nest, when offered sweetened water to drink, chose a mixture of sugar and water that was less sweet.

Cortisol is linked to insulin resistance and deposition of visceral fat (which surrounds abdominal organs and has a toxic effect). Cortisol also drives stress eating.

The simplest way to reduce cortisol is exercise.

Those stress hormones were designed to help us get away from charging animals.

When feeling "stressed out" an excellent thing to do is to get up and move — shake out the kinks, dance around the room, jump up and down.

Meditation is also helpful, particularly for noticing and dropping the kinds of thoughts that lead to anxiety.   — M.S.

GLUCOSE TESTING

Sometimes when I think about the prevalence of prediabetes, my family history, and my past as far as food goes, I am amazed that I've managed to escape.

In fact, after reading more books, articles and blog posts about metabolic impairment than I care to count, I began to wonder if I could have developed the condition since my last screening glucose test.

It's pretty typical for students of medicine to think they have most every disease they learn about. Although well past my student days, I know I have risk factors. Besides, "Inquiring minds want to know." Just because my fasting blood sugar three years ago was under a hundred, didn't mean it had stayed in that range.

That's when I decided to conduct my own one-person experiment. I arranged to get the test done by a lab. Before breakfast I went to have my blood drawn.

Next I headed to the chain drugstore a few blocks away to look at glucose meters. Prices started at just under fifteen dollars, which seemed reasonable given what's at stake. It's the test strips that jack up the cost. One kit had test strips included, so that's the one I got.

Despite more than 20 years of working in hospitals, when it came to testing my own blood at home with a device I had never before held in my hands, the process felt daunting. The directions, spread over three separate sheets of paper, all had diagrams and warnings. Plus there was a booklet I was supposed to read all the way through before starting. And I was starving! I wanted to see how my home test matched up with the fasting blood sugar done at the lab.

I'm not sure how far I would have gotten by myself, but by a strange quirk of fate a friend who has diabetes showed up before I chucked the whole thing. She watched patiently while I read the directions aloud. The hardest part was figuring out how to use the lancet to stick my finger. Unable to watch me struggle any longer,

she showed me how the top came off and then talked me through the rest.

After messing up only two of the ten "free" test strips, I managed to get a result — in the 90s. OK.

Two hours after breakfast I tested again and got another result in the normal range, a sign that I had dodged diabetes. I strongly believe that eating fewer carbs has helped.

Proud of my skill at testing, I began imagining taking my new toy over to people's houses to see if they would let me check their blood.

So far I haven't started going door-to-door performing glucose testing, but I do encourage my friends who haven't had a fasting blood sugar test done lately to get one.   — M.S.

RECOMMENDED

BOOKS

See Annotated Bibliography on page 75.

VIDEO

"Sugar: The Bitter Truth", Robert Lustig, M.D., University of California Television, 2009.

ORGANIZATION

Many people have found support groups helpful in changing their relationship to abusable substances. Programs modeled after Alcoholics Anonymous have been shown to be effective in people whose conditions had previously seemed irreversible. Overeaters Anonymous is one such organization. Local meetings can be found on line.

FOOD AND DRINKS THAT ARE NOT RECOMMENDED

The following information is based, in part, on the guidance for parents provided in Dr. Robert Lustig's book *Fat Chance: Beating the Odds Against Sugar, Processed Foods, Obesity and Disease*. As a pediatrician, I agree wholeheartedly with Dr. Lustig's recommendations to parents about what and what not to feed their children.

If you have children or a weight problem, remove the sugared beverages (including soda *and* fruit juice), as well as flavored yogurt from the house. A glass of orange juice has more sugar than a coca cola. So does a single serving of flavored yogurt. Neither coca cola *nor* these products are recommended.

Breakfast cereals formulated for and marketed to children tend to have sugar as the second or third ingredient, making them more a dessert than a main course. Popular brands of peanut butter have added sugar. Some baby foods and infant formulas have unnecessarily large amounts of added sweeteners.

There is an excellent list of red-, yellow- and green-light foods in Dr. Lustig's book.

SUGAR SUBSTITUTES

When it comes to impact on blood glucose levels, not all sugar substitutes (as with fruits and vegetables) are created equal. Certain sweeteners advertised as having "zero carbs", for example, actually raise blood sugar levels in carbohydrate-sensitive individuals.

Sucralose is a non-caloric sweetener and is mostly indigestible. Interestingly, while the liquid form of sucralose has been shown to have little to no effect on blood sugar in diabetics and prediabetics, the granular form (which is commonly packaged in combination with maltodextrin) can cause an appreciable rise.

Sorbitol, xylitol, and **mannitol** are sugar alcohols. They are frequently found in "sugar-free" candies, chewing gum and desserts. While lower in calories and carbohydrates than regular sugar, some sugar alcohols can significantly raise blood sugar. Large amounts of these substances cause bloating and other intestinal symptoms.

Erythritol, also a sugar alcohol, occurs naturally in certain fruits and fermented foods. It does not affect blood sugar and is less likely to cause gastrointestinal side effects than the other sugar alcohols. None of the sugar alcohols contain the intoxicant ethanol.

Finding out which or whether any sweetener is right for a given individual requires personal investigation. For some, the range of options with regard to sweeteners and desserts is wider than for others. This is, in part, determined by genetics and influenced by environmental factors beginning with the *in utero* environment.

The most direct way to determine the effect of a sugar substitute is, of course, to test blood sugar before and two hours after ingesting the substance. A less exact, but helpful method is to take note of whether ingesting a particular sugar substitute leads to cravings or a compulsion to eat more than intended.

Given the unquestionably serious consequences of high blood sugars in people with impaired metabolism, using a sugar substitute may provide a safer option than eating a dessert sweetened with table sugar, agave, honey, or other caloric, carbohydrate-rich substances. Keep in mind that a cup of tea, a small handful of almonds or a serving of berries also make excellent alternatives to more traditional desserts.

ANNOTATED BIBLIOGRAPHY

Bays, Jan Chosen, M.D. *Mindful Eating: A Guide to Rediscovering a Healthy and Joyful Relationship with Food.* Boston: Shambhala Publications, Inc., 2009.

Dr. Bays, who is a Zen master and a pediatrician, has written a beautiful book describing practices for being more fully present with the pleasures of eating. She discusses seven kinds of hunger including visual hunger and heart hunger.

Bernstein, Richard K., M.D. *Dr. Bernstein's Diabetes Solution: A Complete Guide to Achieving Normal Blood Sugars*, Revised and Updated. New York: Little, Brown and Company, 2011.

Dr. Bernstein's internationally acclaimed program is based on good nutrition, healthy exercise and (where necessary) small doses of medication. His low carbohydrate solution has helped patients of all ages (those with type 1 and type 2 diabetes) achieve normal blood sugars. His book includes case studies of patients who have experienced remarkable improvements in their diabetes when they followed his low-carbohydrate recommendations.

Dr. Bernstein, following his own program, has been living well with type 1 diabetes for 64 years.

Lustig, Robert, M.D. *Fat Chance: Beating the Odds Against Sugar, Processed Food, Obesity, and Disease.* New York: Hudson Street Press, 2013.

Robert Lustig, M.D., is a pediatric neuroendocrinologist, and professor of clinical pediatrics at the University of California, San Francisco.

Dr. Lustig's work goes a very long way toward dispelling the myth that "gluttony and sloth" are what has caused the obesity epidemic. If anyone can explain in clear and convincing terms the toxicity of sugar, it is Dr. Lustig. His video "Sugar: the Bitter Truth," has, to date, been viewed nearly four million times. The fact that it covers a 1½-hour lecture on metabolism gives an idea of how compelling and entertaining Dr. Lustig's explanations can be. Everyone with an interest in health, especially children's health, is encouraged to read *Fat Chance*. The clinical vignettes are powerfully illustrative. The science is impeccable.

Nestle, Marion, M.D. *Food Politics: How the Food Industry Influences Nutrition and Health*, Revised and Expanded Tenth Anniversary Edition.[1] London: University of California Press, 2013.

Dr. Nestle's award winning book *Food Politics* was under attack by food industry representatives even before it was published. According to author and activist Michael Pollan, *Food Politics* is "one of the founding documents of the movement to reform the American food system."[2] Marion Nestle, Ph.D., M.P.H. is professor of Nutrition, Food Studies and Public Health at New York University.

Parker, Steve, M.D. *Conquer Diabetes and Prediabetes: The Low-Carb Mediterranean Diet.* Phoenix: pxHealth, 2011.

Steve Parker, M.D., has over two decades' experience practicing Internal Medicine treating patients with diabetes and prediabetes. He is an expert on the Mediterranean diet. Dr. Parker offers a modification of this diet, called the Ketogenic Mediterranean diet, for people who are insulin resistant. Helping them to understand in clear language how they differ in their ability to metabolize carbohydrates, Dr. Parker offers a livable, accessible and effective way to lower circulating blood sugar and maintain good health despite these conditions. Including specific recommendations for meals and recipes, *Conquer Diabetes and Prediabetes* is an invaluable nutritional guide for all those struggling to maintain healthy blood sugar levels.

Peeke, Pam. *The Hunger Fix.* New York: Rodale, 2012.

The Hunger Fix is Dr. Peeke's *New York Times* best-selling book about food addiction. Her description of the effects of binge eating on dopamine receptors[3] offers insight into what people with eating disorders are up against. The book offers many practical suggestions for replacing "false fixes," such as food obsession and overeating, with healthier rewards.

Taubes, Gary. *Why We Get Fat and What To Do About It.* New York: Anchor Books, 2010.

Gary Taubes has received three Science in Society Journalism awards, the only print journalist to do so. He is contributing correspondent for *Science* magazine and recipient of a Robert Wood Johnson Foundation Investigator award in Health Policy Research at the University of California,

---

[1] The book was written prior to important discoveries about the respective roles of dietary fat and carbohydrates, but remains a classic.

[2] In the forward to the 2013 revised edition of *Food Politics*.

[3] Dopamine receptors are found in the central nervous system and appear to have a crucial role in pleasure, motivation, and neuroendocrine signaling.

Berkeley School of Public Health. In his book *Why We Get Fat and What To Do About It*, Mr. Taubes writes about the history and politics of science, in particular, research into the causes of obesity, in ways that are "un-put-downable." ***Why We Get Fat*** challenges paradigms that need challenging. Its content makes sense of the multiplicity of factors contributing to the diabetes and obesity epidemics. Mr. Taubes' writing helps readers understand the impact that refined carbohydrates have on weight and health.

ABOUT THE AUTHORS

CONSTANCE HOLMES, ED.D

Constance Holmes was trained as a psychologist in the Child Psychiatry Service at Massachusetts General Hospital, a Harvard training institution, from 1975-1982. She received her doctorate from Boston University in 1981 and was licensed in Massachusetts in 1982. She relocated to Berkeley, CA in 2000 and was granted her California license in 2002.

Dr. Holmes has worked with cancer patients and their families in hospitals, inpatient and outpatient clinics and within non-profit cancer support organizations for 25 years. An experienced group leader as well as a conference presenter, she has published several articles in oncology journals on issues relating to end-of-life care.

MARTHA SNIDER, M.D.

As a pediatrician, one of Martha Snider's favorite tasks was counseling parents on the care and feeding of infants and children. During her clinical career she was chair of a 30-person department and assistant chief of a 260-bed hospital. For more than a decade, she has worked as a consultant to the Medical Board of California, an agency whose mission is to protect the public health and safety.

As a certified Rosen Method movement teacher, she has taught range-of-motion exercise classes in health facilities and community centers.

Her paintings, photographs and collages have been exhibited at the Women's Cancer Resource Center in Oakland, California; Picturish Gallery in Berkeley, California, and the Oakland Public Library.

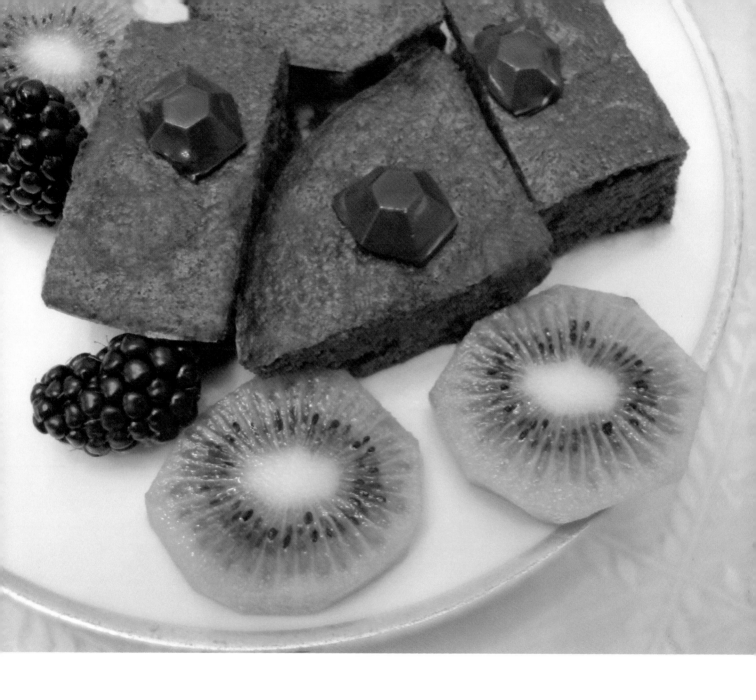

NOTES

CPSIA information can be obtained
at www.ICGtesting.com
Printed in the USA
LVIC06n2244120114
369152LV00001B/1

9781587902529